Adventures in Blood

Adventures in Blood

The Quest for Safe Blood and
a Universal Cure

Dr. Ehud Ben-Hur

To order additional copies of this book, contact:
Xlibris Corporation
1-888-795-4274
www.Xlibris.com
Orders@Xlibris.com
68620

CONTENTS

Lux et Vita

ACKNOWLEDGEMENTS

I WOULD LIKE to thank the following friends whose comments during the preparation of this book helped improve its accuracy. Drs. Bernard Horowitz, Richard Shulman, Ionel Rosenthal, Tom Dubbelman, Eli Heldman and Tom Petrie. Special thanks are due to my wife Dina for editorial comments and for my son Adi who designed the front cover.

ACKNOWLEDGMENTS

INTRODUCTION

R ECENTLY I RETIRED (more or less) to Fort Collins, CO, a quiet university town on the Northern Front Range. During that period I had time to reflect on recent events of my life. I decided there was enough public interest to justify an effort to try and write it up in an accessible form and this slim book is the result.

I was born in Israel (the British mandate of Palestine at the time) in 1940, on a farming community (kibbutz Kineret) located on the southern tip of the Sea of Galilee. My parents (David and Miriam) were young pioneers at the time. They emigrated in the mid 1930 from Eastern Europe with the aspiration for a new life without anti-Semitism. At the age of 10 I already knew I was going to be a scientist and focused since then on becoming one. It took 20 years. At the age of 30 I obtained my doctorate diploma in Chemistry from the Technion (Israel Institute of Technology). During the intervening years my life was quite normal for an Israeli at that period. At age 18 I did my tour of duty in the army (Corps of Engineers). I served for 2.5 years and was discharged with the rank of lieutenant. During my service I met my future wife Dina, whom I married before graduating from the Hebrew University. I served one month a year during the ensuing 30 years as a reservist in the army, studied hard the rest of the time, and did research for my thesis.

As a newly minted scientist (specializing in biochemistry of nucleic acids) I went for a postdoctoral stint at Brookhaven National Laboratory in New York. There I did basic research on the biological effects of various radiations at the lab of Dr Mortimer Elkind, a world renowned expert in radiation biology. I returned to Israel in 1973 as an Assistant Professor at the Hebrew University, just in time to participate in my second war, the Yom Kippur one. A couple of years later I was tempted to join the Radiation Biology Department of the Nuclear Research Center—Negev, where I continued basic research studies of radiation effects on biological systems.

The above experience prepared me only to some extent for the adventures, to be described in this slim volume. It was the confluence of quite a few lucky events that caused me at the ripe age of 52 to embark on a new and thrilling scientific adventure. While the story is mostly linear in time, some breaks are taken to describe the relevant science that underlies the events.

CHAPTER 1

OUT OF ISRAEL

TOWARDS THE END of the nineteen eighties, the interest in my research by the powers that be at the Nuclear Research Center-Negev (NRCN) was waning. This research was focused at that time on photodynamic treatment (PDT). It was spurred by the Lasers Department upon my return from a sabbatical year in Colorado State University in 1983. At the time, medical applications for a new laser (copper vapor laser and later gold vapor laser) were sought by the Lasers Department. The combination of this laser with an appropriate photosensitizer for use in PDT was deemed a worthwhile pursuit.

PDT was then an experimental approach to cancer treatment. PDT utilizes the tendency of certain dyes to localize in tumors. The localized dye is activated by laser light of an appropriate wavelength. Light exposure produces reactive oxygen species (ROS) which eradicate the tumor. Initially it was thought that the disappearance of the tumor was the result of direct kill of the tumor cells. Now we know that shutting off blood circulation to the tumor is largely responsible for its elimination.

PDT is now an established modality for the treatment of certain types of cancer as well as age-related macular degeneration, the leading cause of blindness in the elderly. For an overview of PDT see the cancer society website: www.cancer.org/docroot/ETO/content/ETO_1_3x_Photodynamic_Therapy.asp

Shortly after initiating the PDT studies I found that some of the phthalocyanines, a class of dyes used widely in industry, are potent photosensitizers with a marked affinity to tumors. Phthalocyanines (Pc) are porphyrin-like blue dyes. Their advantage for use in PDT was their strong absorption of light in the red, a portion of the spectrum where light penetration into tissue is maximal. These findings were soon followed up by a number of other groups but the interest in it at NRCN dropped for reasons that had nothing to do with science. As a result, I took another sabbatical year in 1990 to pursue my studies at the medical school of Leiden

University, Holland, with Dr Tom Dubbelman. Tom was leading a group studying the mechanism of action of PDT. I first met Tom in 1984 during a PDT meeting in Sardinia and he struck me as a gentle and intelligent guy and an excellent scientist.

The Netherlands proved to be the opposite of Israel in most respects. The weather is mostly cloudy, the country flat and green and water is abundant. I rented a house in a small town near Leiden that was situated on a major canal. It was pleasure watching the traffic on the canal and sailing on it with my neighbor. The people were kind, helpful and relaxed. This, together with excellent facilities allowed me to pursue my work most effectively and publish a few papers. One of them was a breakthrough of sorts and another study focused on the ability of Pc to kill viruses when exposed to red light. This property triggered the idea that it could reduce pathogens in blood, thus reducing the risk of transmitting these pathogens during blood transfusion.

Upon returning to Israel at the end of 1991 I received a letter from Dr. Bernard Horowitz, Vice President at the NY Blood Center (NYBC). Dr. Horowitz was also the Head of the Virus Inactivation Laboratory at NYBC and has recently developed and commercialized a process to inactivate viruses in plasma and blood proteins. Because the process used a detergent it could not be used for the cellular components of blood (red cells and platelets) because the detergent would dissolve the cell membrane. To sterilize the cellular components he focused on the use of light-activated dyes such as Pc. Dr Horowitz praised my work and extended an invitation to visit the NYBC. Likewise he invited me to present my work at a Symposium on virus inactivation in blood he was organizing at the American Society of Photobiology annual meeting in Florida during the next summer. I gave my consent and in June of 1992 met Dr. Horowitz in Florida. Bernie, as he insisted to be called, proved to be a tall, charming guy with twinkling intelligent eyes. During the meeting we had dinner with two of his colleagues. One was Shanti, a petite west-Indian girl, the other a blonde by the name of Henrietta. Both nice enough girls but dwarfed by their imposing boss. Afterward Bernie asked if I would consider joining NYBC to head his lab, as his VP duties interfered with his effective management in the lab. I said I was honored and will seriously consider his offer after returning to Israel and consulting my wife.

I found my wife unenthusiastic about the move. Leaving behind two grown boys, newly custom built house and a bunch of good friends tipped the balance for staying. Nevertheless, she was willing to consider the move and in October we visited NYBC for further discussions, following which I gave my consent. Upon returning to Israel I tended my resignation to the NRCN, effective the end of the year. My Department arranged for a farewell party during which I said goodbye to my colleagues, some of them were sorry to see me go. I had no second thoughts and was quite excited about the prospects in the New World. Later we had a farewell party at home, where family and friends saw me off. In February of 1993 I arrived in NYC. Dina, could not join me right away since my younger son, Adi, was still serving in the army and leaving him by himself at such time was not an option. She decided to come after his discharge and the start of his studies for graphic design later in the autumn.

Before describing my adventures in the big apple and the pursuit of a safer blood, some background information on blood is needed for the reader's edification.

CHAPTER 2

BLOOD—MYTHS AND FACTS

B LOOD HELD A special place in human consciousness over the eons. It was thought to contain the life force, since the loss of a large amount of blood led to death. According to the Bible: "The blood is the soul". It is first mentioned in the Bible with regard to the first murder. God's voice asks Cain: "What hast thou done? The voice of your brother's blood cried unto me from the ground".

Red, the color of blood, was thought to have magical powers. Early Egyptians painted their bodies with blood to avert disease. Later, dyes were substituted for this practice, leading eventually to makeup. In England, red coverings on bed were used to combat smallpox and red cloth as a cure for scarlet fever.

According to one myth, a corpse could identify its assassin by bleeding. This dates back to the murder of King Henry II. While Richard, his son, approached the body, the dead King allegedly had a nose-bleed.

The preponderance of vampires in many cultures is another indication to our fascination with blood. Again, the ability of blood to invest the vampire with supernatural powers attests to the magical potency ascribed to blood.

These and many other myths about blood have mostly disappeared nowadays but some remain and interfere with medical practice. In certain rural areas it is believed that removal of vital spirits residing in the blood during the taking of blood samples, affects our health adversely. As a result, these people avoid this necessary procedure.

Bloodletting by phlebotomy has been an obsession with medical practitioners for thousands of years, causing countless suffering. Initially this was done for unproven indications and more recently for diagnostic purposes. Since the 19th century progress has been made in spite of considerable opposition from the medical establishment. Today, the only indication for bloodletting is in the case of hemochromatosis, where there is overproduction of red cells.

The first scientific explanation for the role of blood was offered in the 17th century by Dr. William Harvey. His achievement was the description of the circulation of blood in the human body. In 1710, 53 years after Harvey's death, the English clergyman Stephen Hales demonstrated blood pressure in the circulation in a dramatic manner. He attached a glass tube to an artery of a horse and watched blood rise to a height of 8 feet 3 inches. The first working model of the circulatory system was devised by a German physician in 1677 and the 18th century witnessed the creation of 'blood machines' of increasing sophistication.

A review of our current knowledge of blood is out of the scope of this book. Instead, a basic understanding of blood will be provided to enable the reader to follow the book's themes.

Blood is our inner sea, formed during the evolution of complex organisms that could no longer derive their nutritional needs directly from the surrounding water. Indeed, the salty taste of blood as a result of its high salt content is a remnant of this heritage.

The functions of blood

Broadly speaking, blood has two main functions: to supply the cells of our body with their nutritional needs and to remove the byproducts of their metabolism. In addition, the blood contains major elements of the immune system. It also serves as a delivery system of hormones, allowing communication between distant organs.

Delivery of oxygen from the lungs to the cells to support respiration and removing carbon dioxide, the byproduct of respiration, is a major function of blood. This is accomplished by the red blood cells. Other nutrients—essential amino acids, vitamins, sugar, lipids and minerals—are delivered in a soluble form or bound to specific blood proteins.

Blood clotting is a vital property of blood, designed to prevent its loss in the event of a breach of the circulatory system. The clotting process is very complex and is carried out by a number of proteins and specialized small cells—platelets. The clotting proteins act in a highly orchestrated manner and interact with the platelets to form a blood clot. When any one of these components is absent or malfunctions a severe bleeding disorder results.

The composition of the blood

Blood volume in an average person is about 5 liters or about 7% body weight. It is composed of a variety of cells suspended in a water solution of proteins and small organic molecules as well as salts. Broadly speaking, blood cells are divided into red cells, platelets and white cells.

Red cells. Red cells comprise close to half of the blood volume. Blood hematocrit (the percentage of blood volume made up by red cells) is usually 40-50. The mature red cell is a membrane sac full of hemoglobin—the oxygen carrier molecule. Hemoglobin is composed of a protein moiety—globin, and heme—a porphyrin molecule with the oxygen binding iron atom at its center. The heme component absorbs blue light strongly, hence its red color. Venous blood reaching the lungs is low in oxygen and has a high affinity to it. The opposite is the case for arterial blood reaching the capillaries supplying the tissues. As a result, oxygen binds to hemoglobin in the lungs and is released where it is needed. Hemoglobin changes color from deep to bright red upon oxygen binding. This is the basis for measuring oxygen saturation of blood in medical practice.

Carbon dioxide, generated in tissues as a byproduct of cell respiration, diffuses into the blood and is converted to bicarbonate. In this soluble form it is delivered by the plasma to the lungs, where it is released as a gas due to the difference in its concentrations between blood and air.

Red cells, unlike most other cells, contain no nucleus and thus have no nucleic acids. Their discoid shape is also unique among cells, which are spheroid when suspended in liquid. Their unique shape, together with their ability to deform, allows their easy passage through the blood capillaries, the diameter of which is somewhat smaller than that of the red cell.

The red cells (erythrocytes) are produced from erythroid cells, which in turn are produced in the bone marrow from stem cells and are then released to the circulation. The life-span of the mature red cell in the circulation is about 120 days. Upon their demise they are metabolized in the liver. The rate of production of new red cells is closely controlled by the hormone erythropoietin.

Platelets. Platelets (thrombocytes) are very small cells that are formed from the fragmentation of a large cell, the megakariocyte. They are highly specialized, containing no nucleus, and have only one function: to participate in the process of blood clotting. They do so by adhering to the inner part of blood vessels, the endothelium, at the site of damage, forming the initial plug. This plug is further strengthened by a cascade of protein reactions, leading to the conversion of soluble fibrinogen into insoluble fibrin fibers. Normally, there are 200,000-500,000 platelets in a

DR. EHUD BEN-HUR

microliter of blood. When this number falls below 20,000 blood clotting is impaired.

White cells. The number of white cells in a microliter of blood is 5000-11000. This number increases in case of infectious diseases. They are divided into leukocytes and lymphocytes and each of these is further divided into subgroups according to their structure and function. All the white cells are part of the immune system, participating in highly specialized fights against external invaders. Sometimes, in the case of autoimmune diseases they mistakenly attack body organs.

Plasma. Plasma is the liquid portion of the blood. It has an amber color and is a water solution of thousands of different proteins, most of them in very small amounts, comprising 7% of plasma weight. Albumin is the most abundant protein in plasma (3.5-5 gram in 0.1 liter). It binds myriad compounds for delivery purposes. Immunoglobulins (antibodies) are present at about 1-1.5 gram per 0.1 liter. They are an important part of the immune system. Fibrinogen, the protein that forms blood clots, is the third abundant protein (0.2-0.45 gram per 0.1 liter). Among the small molecules, sugar, lipids (in various forms) and amino acids are relatively abundant and sodium chloride is the major salt. Its concentration is constant at 0.9%.

CHAPTER 3

THE NEW WORLD

I ARRIVED IN NYC on a beautiful crisp winter day and was accommodated at a furnished apartment on York Avenue and 63rd street—a residential complex owned by the Rockefeller University. The NYBC, located 10 min walk away on 67th street, leased some of these apartments to house senior scientists.

In the US half the blood is supplied by blood centers affiliated with the American Red Cross (ARC). The rest is provided by private blood centers. Of the latter, the NYBC is the largest, supplying about 10% of the nation's blood to 250 hospitals. NYBC is located at a number of sites in the metropolitan area, the 67th street location serves as headquarters and the site of its Research Institute. The latter is comprised of about 15 laboratories, spread over 4 floors, that cover most research areas related to blood. The top floor is where the administration resides. NYBC employs about 2000 people and its annual budget is about $300 M.

The following morning I arrived at the blood center, a squat 4 floors building with a white-painted brick façade, and was shown to my department. My small kingdom consisted of 3 labs, each manned by a scientist and a lab technician. The red cells lab was headed by Dr Shanti Rywkin, the platelets lab by Dr Henrietta Nunno, and Dr Bolanle Williams was in charge of the viral assays lab.

Upon meeting with Bernie I found out that the most pressing task was the submission of a grant proposal to the National Institutes of Health (NIH). A previous proposal did not score sufficiently high and was sent back for revision. The deadline for submission was in 2 weeks. It should be noted that research at NYBC is mostly supported by outside grants, so getting the revised proposal out was vital. After a meeting with the lab personnel I immersed myself in this task and sent the proposal on time. While burdensome, it forced me to master all the project details right away and helped in preparing me for the job ahead.

The daily operation of my group was run by the above mentioned scientists. They conducted experiments with their assistants. Every week a meeting of all the scientists was held during lunch time on Monday. Professor Nick Geacintov of NY University was usually present at those meetings. Nick is an expert in photochemistry who first suggested to Bernie the use of Pc for the red cells project and became a consultant for the project. At the meeting each scientist presented the results obtained from experiments conducted during the previous week. This was followed by discussion and finally a recommendation on the best way to proceed. In addition to the weekly meeting I met with the various members of the group as the need arose.

I soon became aware that scientific aspects of the job were only one of the challenges I faced. The suitability of the scientists was another. It was obvious that Dr Williams was not up to the job of introducing new procedures we needed in order to continue with the project. Fortunately, I found that human resources was very helpful and in short order I had been able to replace him with Dr Paul Gottlieb, a brilliant virologist from the nearby Hunter College.

The second personnel problem, one that took much longer to resolve was a bitter rivalry between Shanti and Henrietta. Shanti was the more junior, on a postdoctoral fellowship, while Henrietta was an Assistant Member of the NYBC Research Institute, academically equivalent to an Assistant Professor. None had tenure. While the fact that each worked on a different project reduced the friction, some cooperation was needed when using the common facilities of the viral assays lab. As time went on I became convinced that Shanti's stature as a scientist did not warrant advancing her to an Assistant Member position. As a result, she had to leave when her appointment expired at the end of the year. Meantime our revised grant proposal to the NIH was approved and I decided to restructure the group. I took direct responsibility for the red cells project and hired a Polish analytical chemist, Dr Magda Zuk, whom I knew from her postdoctoral work at North Carolina State University in Raleigh. Magda established an analytical chemistry lab to deal with the chemical aspects of the project.

For the red cell project the aim was to identify a Pc that when activated by red light would eliminate all pathogens with minimal damage to the red cells. My approach was based on screening of a large number of Pc, supplied by Prof. Malcolm Kenney at Case Western Reserve University. Mac is one of the most respected Pc chemists worldwide. We became acquainted during a presentation I gave in Cleveland on the use of Pc in

PDT. Following my talk, Prof. Nancy Oleinick, the head of the Radiation Biology Department, initiated a collaborative program on the subject with Mac, from which I benefited by having an access to their Pc library.

The screening of Pc for our purpose involved 2 steps. First they were tested for their efficacy in killing viruses in red cells when exposed to red light. The active ones were then tested for collateral damage to the red cells. Within a few months of this screening we identified a silicon Pc derivative that Mac has termed Pc4. Pc4 proved to be highly effective against all the viruses tested. Its damage to red cells, while significant, could be potentially eliminated by certain techniques that will be described later.

Before going any further into the development of our 2 projects (for red cells and platelets) some additional background information is needed with respect to blood transfusion and blood safety.

CHAPTER 4

BLOOD TRANSFUSION

THE TRANSFUSION OF blood components or blood products is done in a variety of cases. In each case the blood component transfused is tailored to the patient's need. In case of severe blood loss during trauma or surgery or in patients with blood diseases such as thalasemia and sickle cell anemia, red cells are transfused. For thrombocytopenia (a disease where platelets are in severe shortage) or in cancer patients undergoing chemotherapy, transfusion of platelets takes place. Hemophiliacs, in whom certain clotting factors are deficient, obtain clotting factors.

The science of blood transfusion became possible in the early 19th century due to the discovery of the major blood groups A and B. In the 20th century the Rh group was discovered. This group is important in pregnancy when the mother is negative and the fetus is positive. In such a case during the first pregnancy no adverse effects are evident. The antibodies to the fetus red cells the mother produces can result in hemolytic anemia in the next pregnancy in which the fetus is Rh positive. Other minor blood groups are now known that are not routinely important for blood transfusion. All these groups are determined by certain sugars, protruding from the red cell membrane, that serve as antigens. The O group red cells do not carry these sugars and can be transfused to people carrying any other group. The AB group carries the antigens of both A and B and can receive blood from all other groups but donate only to AB. Any mismatch of these major groups during blood transfusion can be fatal.

Initially, only direct transfusion from donor to recipient was performed since blood coagulates shortly after storage. In the early 20th century, upon the discovery of anticoagulants, blood storage became feasible. It led eventually to the establishment of blood banks, first the Soviet Union in 1930 and then in the USA in 1937. At that time, whole blood was transfused. During the 1940's the separation of blood into its components by centrifugation was introduced. These components include red cells, platelets and plasma. Each component is stored differently to maximize its storage time. Red cell concentrate is stored refrigerated (at 1-6 degrees centigrade) for up to 6 weeks, platelets are stored at room temperature with continuous shaking for up to 5 days and plasma can be kept frozen at -80 degrees centigrade for years. In the 1950's plastic bags were substituted for storage instead of glass bottles. This greatly facilitated blood separation and storage and allowed blood banking to move from individual hospitals to regional blood centers, where most blood collection and distribution is done nowadays.

As of 2005 about 15 million blood units were transfused in the US, mostly red cells (about 12 million) and the rest platelets and plasma. The latter is used in case of coagulation diseases. Blood products are proteins derived from plasma, such as coagulation factors used for hemophiliacs, albumin and immunoglobulins. The coagulation factors are now produced also by the biotech industry using recombinant technologies.

During the last 30 years attempts were made to produce oxygen-carrying substitutes to red cells. These attempts are mostly based on hemoglobin from either animal or human sources. So far none of the modified hemoglobins was approved for human use although one product is used in veterinary practice. The driving force for these efforts is manifold. Immediate availability in trauma cases, ease of storage and safety aspects. These efforts are ongoing.

The benefits of transfusion are obvious but they do not come risk-free. The risk of transmitting infectious disease will be discussed in the next chapter. In addition there are risks of human errors when delivering the blood to the patient and some adverse reactions even when using matched blood. Some of these reactions are produced by the white cells. To reduce those reactions the blood can be filtered prior to transfusion (leukoreduction) or irradiated with ionizing radiation (at a dose of 25 Gy) to inactivate the leukocytes.

To obviate some of the risks involved with blood transfusion a patient undergoing a planned surgery can donate and store some blood in advance. This is termed autologous transfusion (homologous transfusion is the term for the common practice). It constitutes only a small fraction of blood transfusion and is not encouraged because it involves additional logistics for the hospital.

CHAPTER 5

TRANSFUSION-TRANSMITTED INFECTIOUS DISEASE

IT HAS LONG been recognized that blood transfusion can transmit infectious diseases. These diseases, most of them caused by viruses, include the following.

Hepatitis C. Caused by hepatitis C virus (HCV). After the initial acute phase some patients are able to clear the virus but in many, a chronic phase ensues. During this phase the virus multiplies in the liver and is present in the blood at a level that can vary by orders of magnitudes among individuals, but is relatively constant in each person. The chronic phase can last years and eventually leads to liver fibrosis and cirrhosis. In about a quarter of the patients liver cancer may result. It is estimated that in the US about 4 million are infected.

Hepatitis B. The disease manifestation is similar to that of hepatitis C. The causative agent (HBV) is a DNA virus rather than the RNA virus that cause hepatitis C. Because a vaccine is available against HBV, it is not prevalent in the US but in the Far East it is endemic.

Hepatitis A. The hepatitis A virus (HAV) causes an acute infection of the liver. The infection is resolved and no virus remains in the circulation within a few weeks. Its transmission by transfusion is therefore very rare. However, because fresh frozen plasma can be pooled for processing and blood products are produced by pooling of thousands of plasma units, transfusion of these products can result in a higher frequency of transmission.

Human T-lymphocytic virus. HTLV (in its 2 forms) infects the lymphocytes and in 1-2% of the cases can lead to leukemia. Its prevalence in the US is low.

AIDS. The AIDS pandemic was first recognized in 1982 as a strange affliction of homosexuals in San Francisco. A year later the causative agent was identified as the human immunodeficiency virus (HIV), a close relative of HTLV. The acute phase after infection has flu-like symptoms. During the chronic phase the virus attacks specific cells of the immune system called helper T cells (designated CD 4). It circulates in the blood as a free virus and inside the T cells and is present in other tissues, notably the semen, hence its ability to be transmitted during sexual intercourse. AIDS was fatal in most cases within 10 years after infection, when the level of CD4 cells dropped very low and opportunistic infections (e.g. bacterial pneumonia) became rampant. Some types of cancer such as Kaposi's sarcoma are also typical of AIDS. Nowadays potent antiviral drugs are available and allow patients to live much longer. In the US there are about 1 million infected individuals (40 million worldwide). The transmission of AIDS by blood transfusion put the spotlight on blood safety and facilitated the introduction of measures to avoid the risk.

West Nile virus. The disease was recently introduced into the US by infected mosquitoes and is prevalent in all the states during the summer. While symptoms in most infected individuals are mild (flu-like), in a small percentage they can be severe and affect the central nervous system. The elderly and people with deficient immune system are particularly at risk. Because there is no chronic phase to the infection the risk to the blood supply is small.

Malaria. This tropical disease is caused by a parasite of the red cells (various Plasmodium species) and is rarely transmitted by blood transfusion in the US. Travelers to countries where the disease is endemic can get infected and carry the parasite back home. Because of global warming, infections transmitted by the vector (a mosquito), originating in the US were recorded.

Chagas' Disease. The causative agent is the parasite *Trypanosoma cruzi* and it is endemic in Latin America (about 20 million infected). The disease is chronic and can lead to enlarged heart and death. The parasite is present in the blood at low levels and is transmitted by an insect that is present in adobe dwellings. Because of the large immigrant population from Latin America in the US, transmission during blood transfusion can occur.

Syphilis. This sexually transmitted disease is caused by a bacterium that is present in the blood. The last recorded transmission as a result of blood transfusion was in the 1960's.

Mad cow disease. This bovine disease, is caused by an unusual infectious agent, a protein called *prion.* In humans, a similar disease that is invariably fatal is termed Creutzfeld-Jacobs syndrome and is very rare. Mad cow disease can be transmitted to humans by eating infected cows. The disease can be transmitted by blood transfusion.

Prevention

In order to reduce the risk of transmission of infectious disease during blood transfusion a number of steps were instituted in the developed countries.

Deferral. Prior to donating blood the donor is asked questions related to his lifestyle and travel history. People who engage in homosexual activity or traveled recently to countries where malaria is endemic are deferred from donation. The same holds true for those who lived for more than 6 months during the last few years in England, where mad cow disease has spread during the 1990's.

Screening. In the US all donated blood is screened by testing for the following diseases: AIDS, hepatitis B, Hepatitis C, HTLV, West Nile virus and syphilis. Blood that is tested positive is discarded. Testing was done in the past by looking for antibodies produced in response to the infectious agent. The problem with this approach is that it takes a few weeks after infection before a detectable level of antibodies is reached. During this window period the infected donated blood can transmit the disease after transfusion. To shorten the window period, a nucleic acid technology (NAT) was implemented for testing HIV, HCV, HBV and WNV in recent years. The NAT tests for the presence of the virus nucleic acid in the blood. It is sensitive enough to detect the virus a few days after infection. As a result, the risk of transfusing an infected blood unit was reduced 10-fold, from about 1 in 100,000 to 1 in a million.

In the rare cases when skin bacteria are introduced into the blood during donation, they can multiply in platelet concentrates during storage at room temperature and cause morbidity and even mortality in the transfused patients. This poses no problem for red cells that are stored in the cold. Screening methods for the presence of bacteria in platelets were developed but are effective in only about 80% of the cases.

CHAPTER 6

PATHOGEN REDUCTION IN BLOOD: INTRODUCTION

I ADDITION TO deferral and detection, reduction of pathogens present in blood for transfusion is another way to prevent transmission of disease during transfusion. This was first attempted in 1940's when pooling of plasma during World War II was recognized as a source of hepatitis. Treatment with short wave ultraviolet light (UVC) could inactivate the causative virus but the dose needed reduced the activity of clotting factors in the plasma.

The next impetus for pathogen reduction in blood for transfusion was the advent of the AIDS pandemic. The possibility of contamination is particularly acute in blood products made from pooled plasma, because the risk of pathogen transmission is directly proportional to the number of pooled units (for a pool made of 1000 units the risk is 1000 times higher). As a result, such products were the first to be available in sterile form. However, before this has been accomplished in 1985 thousands of hemophiliac patients were infected with HIV and HCV. In France officials did not adopt sterilization technology developed in the US immediately when it became available and instead waited a few months until a French version was developed. This caused the infection of hundreds of additional patients and a scandal that resulted in arrests and conviction of some of those involved.

Various methods are available to achieve pathogen reduction in blood products: wet and dry heat, UVC, low pH, nanofiltration and the treatment with solvent and detergent. The latter technology, basically a washing procedure, was developed at NYBC by Dr. Horowitz and is particularly effective. A few hours treatment with solvent and detergent at room temperature guarantees inactivation of any amount of lipid enveloped viruses. This covers all the major risk factors: HIV, HTLV, HBV and HCV. Because the minor viruses that are not lipid-enveloped (HAV and parvo virus B19), are not inactivated, treatment with solvent/detergent of blood products is combined with a second inactivation technique.

The effectiveness of pathogen reduction is measured in logarithms (logs) on the basis of 10. Each log represents a factor of 10. Thus, 5 log reduction means 100,000-fold reduction. To ensure that a treatment reduces sufficient amount of virus in a blood unit to make it virus-free, at least 7 log inactivation has to take place.

While development and adoption of pathogen reduction technologies for blood products was relatively fast, this was not the case for blood components, particularly the cellular blood components, red cells and platelet concentrates. This is because cells are more complex and fragile than proteins. The harsh methods adequate for the latter are destructive for the former. Fresh-frozen plasma (FFP) was the only blood component for which the treatment with the solvent/detergent technology proved adequate early on and was approved for use. The efforts to achieve success for red cells and platelets will be described in the next few chapters.

CHAPTER 7

PATHOGEN REDUCTION IN PLATELET CONCENTRATES—I

BECAUSE PLATELETS DO not contain nucleic acids the efforts to develop a process to reduce pathogens in platelet concentrates have focused on chemicals that target nucleic acids and are activated by light. The use of light allow a precise control of the extent of the chemical reaction. Most of those chemicals were furocoumarins (psoralens), activated by UVA light. The psoralens have been used in dermatology for quite some time to treat the skin disorders vitiligo and psoriasis and their photochemistry is fairly well understood. When added to a biological system psoralens bind to nucleic acids in the dark to form a complex by intercalating between the nucleic acid bases. Upon exposure to light the psoralen absorbs a photon and forms a covalent bond with a nucleic acid base. This monoadduct can absorb another photon of light to form an additional bond with a second nucleic acid base on the complementary chain thus forming a cross-link between the two nucleic acid chains. These cross-links are highly lethal to the virus since they prevent the separation of the chains that is required for their transcription and replication.

The Cerus Corporation and NYBC were the pioneers in pursuing the use of psoralens for pathogen reduction around 1990. Both focused initially on the most effective psoralen known at the time, AMT. Cerus had a number of advantages over NYBC in this pursuit. It had the best psoralen chemists and as a commercial enterprise it could fund the project much better than NYBC. Indeed, since AMT was not ideal for the purpose, Cerus developed a new psoralen termed S-59, with a number of advantages, being more effective and selective than AMT. In addition, it was not mutagenic in the dark and thus was potentially less toxic.

My group at NYBC circumvented the above disadvantages of AMT in 2 ways. First, by using UVA of longer wavelengths and a scavenger of reactive oxygen species (the plant flavonoid quercetin) we eliminated the collateral damage to platelets and made the process highly selective. Second, following treatment the platelets were passed through a filter to remove essentially all the remaining AMT and thus rendering the product non-mutagenic. In spite of the fact that the treated platelets could now be entered into a clinical study to obtain FDA approval for their use in transfusion medicine, an insurmountable obstacle caused us to discontinue the project. It appeared that Cerus had a blocking patent in which they claimed all psoralens as potentially useful for pathogen reduction, including AMT. So unless Cerus granted NYBC the right to do so, NYBC could not commercialize a process based on AMT. In view of their involvement it was highly unlikely Cerus would grant a competitor that right.

As a result, in 1995 we restarted the platelet project from the scratch, looking for a candidate to replace AMT. A short time before, another biotech company, Cryopharm, went bankrupt. Cryopharm started by trying to develop freeze dried platelets to overcome their short shelf life and later extended the effort to include pathogen reduction using compounds similar to the psoralens. Their results did not satisfy their investors who stopped the financing and the company ceased to exist. Before the final dissolution, Cryopharm sold all its assets, physical as well as intellectual, namely their patents. Before describing my involvement in this process, some changes at NYBC affecting my project need to be described.

DR. EHUD BEN-HUR

CHAPTER 8

THE FORMATION OF VITEX

I N 1995 NYBC decided that in order to commercialize the products developed in its research laboratories it had to form an independent company. The company was called VI Technologies, Inc. (VI is short for virus inactivation) or Vitex for short. Into Vitex were transferred certain assets of NYBC such as a plasma fractionation plant at Melville on Long Island. In addition, all the intellectual properties related to pathogen reduction, such as the patents related to the SD-treated plasma and red cells, as well as patents related to the development of a biological glue that could replace suturing during surgery, using fibrinogen and thrombin. The laboratories involved in the development of these products were transferred from NYBC to Vitex. This spin-off involved financing by a private equity firm in return for a substantial portion of the shares in Vitex.

The business model envisaged profits from the plasma fractionation plant supporting the R&D until commercialization of the various projects could be achieved. At some point a public offering was deemed necessary. The major step prior to Vitex becoming a public company was the launch of sterile FFP treated by the SD process.

Soon after its formation, Vitex rented a floor in a newly built biotech building at the Columbia University Medical Complex on 168th street, on the site of the Audubon Theater in which Malcolm X was murdered some 30 years before. The floor Vitex has rented was configured to accommodate the R&D laboratories. This took another year before we could actually move in 1996. The advantage of the new location was an affiliation with the medical school of Columbia University, which provided Vitex for a fee access to its facilities.

Vitex was structured around its 2 sites, the plant in Melville, containing the company headquarters including the finance department and quality control, and the R&D portion in Manhattan. The latter was headed by Bernie and included my lab, the biological glue lab headed by Dr Gerry Marx, a plasma lab headed by Dr David Hammond and a formulation lab headed by Dr Zach Yim. In addition, a group in charge of the clinical studies was headed by Dr. Howard Grossberg and a group in charge of the pilot plant headed by Dr Dick Shulman and Dr John Hamman. At the time, the clinical studies included the fibrin glue and SD-treated plasma. The latter got FDA approval shortly after the formation of Vitex and the challenge was to get an approval for the production in the Melville plant and to extend approval in Canada.

After the purchase of a $10 M filling machine which was installed in an appropriate setting at the Melville plant, and when the logistics of distribution of the product were in place, a final approval for marketing of SD-plasma was granted to Vitex by the FDA. A marketing agreement was then signed with the American Red Cross and preparations were made for an initial public offering. The IPO of about $40 M and a share price of $12 gave the company a market capitalization of about $140 M. Vitex became a public company in 1997 and since then had ups and downs, mostly the latter. Its undoing, to be described later, was the lack of significant market penetration by the SD-plasma product, for reasons that had nothing to do with science and a lot to do with the politics of the blood business.

CHAPTER 9

PATHOGEN REDUCTION IN PLATELET CONCENTRATES—II

A ROUND THE TIME we decided to abandon the use of psoralens (AMT) for pathogen reduction in platelet concentrates, Henrietta's term as an Assistant Member at NYBC approached its conclusion. Either she was to be promoted to an Associate Member or she had to be let go. In reviewing her accomplishments and the NYBC requirements for the next level it became clear to me that she will fail to be approved. As a result we had to let her go and we hired Dr Wai-Shun Chan, an Assistant Professor at Sherbrooke University (Canada), in her stead. Wai-Shun was an expert in the photobiology of Pc and I knew him to be an excellent scientist and a nice person from my previous encounters with him at scientific meetings.

Regarding personnel, it appears that some people can't come to terms with the facts of life. Thus, Shanti could not accept that she was not considered good enough for promotion and sued the NYBC for discrimination (being both a woman and belonging to a minority group). This required both Bernie and myself to waste precious time making depositions. The matter was later dismissed and did not reach a trial. Shanti might have hoped that NYBC would opt for a settlement, however the blood center had a strong case and it did not want to make a precedent.

Shortly after Wai-Shun joined us, the question whether to acquire the Cryopharm patents for pathogen reduction in platelets has come up. In considering the matter the Vitex board asked me to evaluate their portfolio. I flew to Pasadena, CA and met with Dr. Ray Goodrich, Cryopharm's Chief Scientific Officer (CSO), who stayed on to sell off the company's assets. Ray is a very nice person and he showed me where all the files were as well as the remaining equipment that was for sale. It was a sad sight to wander in those empty halls and imagine the scientific activity in them prior to the bankruptcy.

It took me a couple of days to go through the files and ascertain that the technology was far from being ready for clinical studies and its chances for success were slim. I thanked Ray for his help and flew back to NY to prepare my report to the board. Vitex bought a few instruments from Cryofarm but more importantly we were able to recruit their virologist, Dr Aris Lazo, to replace the head of our virus assay lab, Paul Gottlieb, who left for another job. Aris proved very effective in introducing a number of viral assays as well as NAT as quality control for SD-plasma.

Meanwhile, Our efforts to find a substitute for AMT consisted in screening various classes of potentially useful compounds. No promising candidate was identified.

In the meantime, Cerus went full steam ahead with their psoralen candidate S-59, now called amotosalen, and entered clinical studies in the US and Europe. After a few years those studies were successfully completed and Cerus filed for marketing approval. In the US the FDA declined to grant approval and asked to repeat the phase III study. The reason was technical and not due to any failure of the study. It appears that Cerus made some changes to the system designed for marketing and thus it was not identical to the one used in the study. In Europe, on the other hand, there was no such problem and marketing approval was obtained in 2002. Even so, market penetration proved a challenge and only now the Blood Intercept, as the system is called, is being slowly adopted in many European countries. The process involves adding amotosalen to the platelets bag, exposing the bag to UVA light for 3 min and then transferring the platelets into another bag containing a "tea bag" with a compound that absorbs the free amotosalen. The process is very effective in inactivating blood borne viruses, parasites and bacteria. It also kills all the white cells and thus preventing adverse events that can be caused by leukocytes in rare cases.

Meantime, Ray Goodrich joined the R&D arm of Cobe, later merged into Gambro, in Denver, CO. There he continued to pursue pathogen reduction in platelets, and early on focused on the vitamin riboflavin for this purpose. Riboflavin serves as a photosensitizer that binds to nucleic acids and upon light exposure produces reactive oxygen species. The latter oxidize a component of the nucleic acids (guanine) and thus inactivate viruses and other pathogens. Compared to amotosalen, riboflavin has a more favorable toxicology profile but is less effective and less selective. Nevertheless, the company, now called CoridianBCT biotechnologies (a subsidiary of CoridianBCT, Inc), is pursuing a process termed Mirasol based on riboflavin and UVA light. It has completed the clinical studies in Europe and received a CE mark allowing to market the product in Europe, pending approval of each country. The technology can be applied also to plasma and red cells, although in the later poor penetration of UVA light will pose a problem.

CHAPTER 10

VITEX IN ACTION

S HORTLY AFTER THE launch of SD-plasma it became clear that market acceptance of the product is not a given. There were two main reasons. The first was the doubling of the price for SD-treated plasma, compared to FFP, although later this price was discounted. The second was resistance by the regional blood centers not affiliated with the American Red Cross (ARC) to the monopoly of the latter. As a result, they mostly declined to use SD-plasma. In addition the private blood centers tried to introduce a competing product. This was donor-retested FFP which was released for use only after the donor came for a second donation and was tested negative again. This procedure ruled out the possibility of the first test falling within the window period. The product was burdened with logistical problems and never took off, but damaged SD-plasma nevertheless. Finally, a scientific argument was raised against SD-plasma, having to do with its being a pooled product.

The problem with pooling many blood units for processing is that a single unit can contaminate the whole pool. Because the SD process is highly effective against lipid-enveloped viruses such as HIV, HBV and HCV these viruses pose no problem for pooling. However, a contamination of the pool by the non-enveloped viruses HAV and parvovirus B19 can occur occasionally. Although these viruses are not a serious health threat, once you eliminated the serious threats people start to focus on the minor ones.

Vitex addressed this challenge by introducing tests based on Nucleic Acids Technology (NAT) for these minor viruses. These are highly sensitive tests so they can be performed on samples from mini-pools (comprised of pooled small samples taken from individual units) rather than individual units. Only if the mini-pool proves to be contaminated the individual units composing it are tested and the contaminated one eliminated. All this is done prior to the formation of the pool for SD treatment, thus ensuring no units contaminated with HAV or parvovirus are introduced into the process.

Thus, all the scientific-based concerns regarding SD plasma safety were addressed. Nevertheless, market penetration remained limited and the product never achieved wide acceptance. Consequently, the Melville SD-plasma plant operated in the red for about 4 years and was eventually closed. As a result, when a new virus appeared the blood industry was caught unprepared. This was the case of WNV, which was transmitted unabated by transfusion during the first two years after its appearance. Eventually a nucleic acid test was developed and each donated blood unit is now tested, adding to its cost. Had pathogen reduction process been in place this could have been avoided.

A viable company needs diversified line of products, flexible but focused R&D and a few potential products in the pipeline. Vitex's main source of revenue was the plasma fractionation plant which operated profitably and the SD-plasma which did not. The R&D was diversified.

Dr Gerry Marx was in charge of developing a biological glue based on fibrinogen and thrombin. This product was meant to substitute for suturing during surgery and to reduce bleeding. The clinical study launched to get FDA approval used an indication that in hind sight was inappropriate. In the study, fibrin glue application was compared with sutures during carotid artery surgery. The primary endpoint for the study was bleeding. Fibrin glue failed this test. It is likely that blood pressure in the artery was too high for the glue. A contributing factor was the change in formulation midstream without adequate overlap studies by the formulation lab. Another biological glue was then proposed. Albumin, another blood protein, coagulates when heated, bonding with adjacent tissue. Pinpoint application of laser light as a heat source allows for precise biological suture formation.

Dr Eli Heldman, a long time colleague, joined Vitex shortly before fibrin glue was discontinued. When Gerry Marx left not long after this Eli took on the albumin solder project. This was also abandoned later because in order to bring it to the clinical study an appropriate partner could not be found. Eli then joined my group to help with the red cells project.

Dr. David Hammond, who was in charge of the plasma lab, headed the efforts of adding yet another layer of safety to SD-plasma. He used UVC light to eliminate non-enveloped viruses. The pooled SD-plasma was passed in a thin film that was exposed to UVC light. The process achieved adequate kill of non-enveloped viruses but at the cost of unacceptable reduction of clotting factors activities, and was abandoned. The plasma lab pursued also the development of assays for the detection of mad cow disease, which was at its peak in England at the time.

My department focused on virus inactivation in red cell concentrates, studies I have touched on briefly before and will be describe more fully in a subsequent chapter.

All those activities were monitored, reviewed and discussed during weekly meetings. My group held a weekly lunch meeting. During the meetings we evaluated the work done, did course correction if needed and planned strategies for the advancement of the project. Usually, two outside consultants were present, Prof Nick Geacintov, the chemist from NYU, and Sara Lustigman, head of the parasitology lab at NYBC who collaborated with us on inactivating parasites in blood. Bernie's attendance was sporadic.

Every Monday at 8 am a bagel and cream cheese breakfast meeting of all lab directors was held. It was chaired by Bernie and allowed people to keep abreast of their colleagues activities. It was mainly for Bernie's benefit so he could keep in constant touch and provide useful feedback. In addition, it allowed everybody to be on the same page.

There was a quarterly meeting chaired by the CEO at Melville for all the company brass and lab directors. Update on activities and financial status were presented by John Barr, the chief operating officer and the chief financial officer. Lab directors sometimes gave an update on their project. The car pooled ride from Manhattan was an informal bonding experience for us.

Finally, there was an annual meeting of the scientific advisory board. The board consisted of scientists with expertise in the various fields of the R&D activities. During the meeting each lab director presented the status of his projects, current challenges and future plans. In depth discussions ensued. These day-long meetings ended with a jovial dinner in a good restaurant. Of all the meetings this was the most satisfying because of the wide scope of discussions and the forum.

CHAPTER 11

ON THE ROAD

TALKING A LOT is part and parcel of a scientist life. Traveling—sometimes a lot—is another aspect. During my life as a scientist I traveled a lot but never as much as during my work at Vitex.

The most appealing to me were the trips to scientific meetings at which I usually presented some of our findings. In addition it was an opportunity to learn about the latest scientific advancements, to interact with colleagues and hear less scientific tidbits. Meetings are a good opportunity for head-hunting and I tried it when we were short-handed.

Visits to commercial enterprises were of a more practical nature. Bernie and me traveled together during the initial phase and I continued on my own when hands on aspects had to be tackled. Most visits were concerned with joint development of the red cells project, such as the construction of an illumination device or the manufacture of liposomes.

Finally, there were trips to carry out studies at collaborating labs. The most important one was the Naval Blood Research Lab in Boston. At this lab we measured the half-life of baboon red cells in the circulation after treatment with our process. This is a very sensitive way to assess damage to red cells. The response of the baboon red cells had to be tested after every change in the process. As a result, trips to Boston were done routinely every few months. During these trips I met Dr Yair Egozy, a scientist at Haemonetics, with history and interests that overlapped mine and expertise in filters. Yair was doing studies on baboon blood in the course of developing new devices for blood processing. Naturally we found an immediate rapport and kept in touch later on.

Other collaborations were with Case Western Reserve University in Cleveland and at contract research labs for specialized tests. During a visit to such a lab near Washington, DC with my technician we had a car collision and he was hurt. Fortunately, he recovered completely and returned to work. This was the only mishap during all my trips.

CHAPTER 12

PATHOGEN REDUCTION IN RED CELL CONCENTRATES

1. Photochemical approaches.

PATHOGEN REDUCTION IN red cell concentrates (RCC) proved to be a tougher challenge than in platelet concentrates. This is because RCC is opaque to UVA light as well as most of the visible light because hemoglobin strongly absorbs light at these wavelengths. It does not absorb in the red, hence its color. As a result, the approach Cerus used to sterilize platelets does not work for red cells. Nevertheless, because the photochemical approach proved so effective for platelets, efforts were made to extend it to RCC using red light and appropriate photosensitizers, with maximum absorption in the red. These efforts were concentrated at the ARC research center, where the focus was initially on the dye methylene blue, and at NYBC using Pc.

Methylene blue is similar to psoralens in that it binds in the dark to nucleic acids non-covalently. Upon exposure to red light reactive oxygen species are produced and react with the nucleic acid to modify it. The nucleic acid function is thereby impaired. The selectivity of this process derives from the short lifetime of the reactive oxygen species and thus they react only with molecules in the vicinity of their formation. However, the selectivity is not absolute because not all the methylene blue binds to nucleic acids. Thus, there is collateral damage to red cell proteins and some impairment of red cell function. In addition, the dye is unable to inactivate HIV that is localized inside the white cells. The ARC has therefore abandoned the use of methylene blue and developed similar dyes that are more selective to nucleic acids. These dyes appear to cause little damage to red cells during treatment that results in extensive inactivation of many blood borne viruses. The process is still in preclinical studies. One of the problems is scaling it up to treat a whole blood unit rather than a small volume of blood, as is routinely done during the research phase. The obstacle is that though red light is not absorbed by the red cells it is refracted from them and the light does not penetrate more than a few millimeters of RCC. Vigorous stirring and mixing of the RCC is needed to achieve homogenous light exposure. While this is feasible it has to be accomplished in a manner that will not adversely affect the red cells and will be compatible with blood banking processes.

At NYBC the focus was on Pc and this was the reason I was invited to head the project. Some of the Pc are highly effective in photosensitizing the inactivation of viruses and during our screening program we found the silicon Pc derivative, Pc 4 to be the most effective. The problem was that Pc do not have an inherent selectivity to nucleic acids and as a result causes unacceptable collateral damage to red cells by the reactive oxygen species produced in the process. We achieved selectivity by a number of ways.

The use of antioxidants. In the course of our studies we found that a number of antioxidants—agents that neutralize reactive oxygen species—protect the red cells without interfering with virus inactivation by Pc. We therefore added to the process 3 of these agents: manitol, vitamin E and cystein.

Liposomes. Pc 4 is water insoluble and has to be added into the RCC in an appropriate vehicle. One vehicle we explored were liposomes, small lipid vesicles, which release the Pc 4 once added to the RCC. It turned out that the lipids composing the liposomes membrane has a profound effect on the selectivity of the process and thus we were able to select a composition that allowed Pc 4 to be more selective, killing virus and minimizing red cell damage. The reason for the selective uptake of Pc 4 from liposomes to viruses rather than red cells is the composition of the membrane of the red cell is quite different from that of viruses.

Carnitine. Carnitine is a small molecule that participates in the turnover of the red cell membrane. We found that adding carnitine to the treated red cells allowed us to minimize the remaining red cell damage, presumably by enhancing repair of oxidative damage in the red cell membrane.

Scale up. The process we developed for pathogen reduction in RCC was based on the treatment of 3 ml blood in a test tube. The challenge was to scale it up to a RCC unit containing 450 ml. The problems are two-fold. First, providing sufficient amount of light of the proper wavelength (660-680 nm) in a reasonable period. Second, an efficient mixing of the blood during irradiation was needed to obtain a homogenous light exposure. Our first contact to develop the needed prototype was a Canadian company (Efos) that specialized in the use of light emitting medical devices. Efos constructed a prototype equipped with hundreds of small light emitting diodes (emitting intense light in the far red) on both sides of a moving transparent platform on which the blood bag was placed. This ensured homogenous exposure to light of the red cells. The device was cumbersome and required 1 hour of exposure to achieve sufficient pathogen reduction. Following this treatment the blood could be stored in the cold for a few weeks without unacceptable damage shown by using standard in vitro assays (hemolysis etc.). However, the survival of baboon red cells in the circulation was about half that of untreated cells.

A new approach for the scale up was sought that will be less cumbersome, will work faster and will result in red cells of higher quality. On Pall's recommendation we contacted M Systems, an engineering outfit in NJ that specialized in developing medical devices. The approach opted for was the use of a static mixing device. This is an ingenious solution for mixing during flow. The device consisted of a transparent tubing into which a spiral plastic is inserted. This causes the flowing blood to be mixed continuously in a very effective manner. The flowing blood was illuminated with powerful light emitting diodes. This approach yielded very satisfying results. Treatment time was reduced to 15 min, the device was compact and user friendly and treated blood quality was acceptable *in vitro*. Unfortunately, we did not reach in vivo testing because the project was abruptly terminated.

2. Non-photochemical approaches.

The Cerus Corporation approached pathogen reduction in RCC by developing a process that does not depend on light. The chemistry involved is complex, but basically it involves an alkylating agent that binds non-covalently to nucleic acids by intercalation. It contains a reactive side-chain that attaches covalently to the nucleic acid bases. This reactive moiety is attached to the main molecule by a frangible chain that breaks apart once the covalent reaction occurred, releasing the rest of the molecule from the nucleic acid. The reaction is completed in a few hours. The released portion is no longer reactive and is removed from the RCC by an adsorption device. This chemical treatment of the RCC proved highly effective in killing most known pathogens without undue damage to the red cells. The only concern seemed to be the initial high toxicity of the starting chemical but Cerus appeared to have it under control. Indeed, everything seemed to go very well using this approach until it reached Phase 3 in clinical studies, the last and decisive phase. During this study some of the patients undergoing repeated infusions of the treated RCC developed antibodies against these red cells. As a result, the study has been halted and Cerus went to the drawing board. After some tinkering with the formulation it now claims that the problem has been solved and a new Phase 1 clinical study has begun.

Pentose was yet another company that had a similar approach to that of Cerus. They too used an alkylating agent that targets nucleic acids. More about Pentose and its approach in the next chapter.

CHAPTER 13

THE FALL

WHILE I WAS busy trying to get the photochemical approach using Pc 4 to work in RCC, Vitex was fighting for its financial survival. Tom Ostermiller, the original CEO, previously an officer of NYBC, was forced to resign. He was deemed too soft and not up to the tough job of nurturing a fledgling company. He was replaced by John Barr, a former president at Haemonetics, a major company involved in the blood business. The new CEO proved to be tough and ambitious. He signed a collaboration agreement with Pall, another major player in the blood business. Pall's contribution was financial, supporting the R&D effort in the area of pathogen reduction and taking an equity position in Vitex. Being a filter production company they provided technical expertise for the removal of Pc 4 from RCC after the treatment. They introduced us to M Systems that worked on constructing prototype device for the treatment.

John tried to improve the market penetration of SD-plasma by terminating the exclusive agreement with the ARC and launching a marketing campaign. However, the initial momentum was lost and the product's use remained limited. Vitex finally had to concede defeat and withdrew SD-plasma from the market. The only remaining bright light was the plasma fractionation activity. This activity became profitable and supplied a stream of cash.

Shortly after the FDA approved the commercial launch of SD-plasma, Vitex took the opportunity and became a public company with an IPO at a share price of $12, raising about $40 MM. The stock went up later to 18 at the maximum but as the initial promise proved to be elusive it then went down below 12.

Meantime our efforts to optimize the red cells treatment process were gaining ground. Initial studies in baboons (performed at the Naval Blood Research Lab in Boston) demonstrated a good recovery of the cells after treatment and we scheduled a meeting with the FDA to present the process and hear their comments, particularly with regard to what additional preclinical studies may be needed prior to initiating phase I clinical studies. Our reception was encouraging, in that the FDA was quite happy with our use of nontoxic chemicals, in contrast to Cerus. While some additional studies were envisaged, we could clearly see a route to clinical studies in about a year.

During that period it became apparent that John was pursuing an alternative path for RCC pathogen reduction. He began talks with Pentose about adopting their technology for this purpose. Pentose was using alkylating agents termed Inactines that targeted nucleic acids, similar to the Cerus process. The Inactines were inferior to the compound used by Cerus from a number of view-points. To begin with. Inactines were less effective and as a result much higher concentration and longer treatment time were needed. Even more alarmingly inactines did not degrade spontaneously and had to be removed after treatment by extensive washing of the RCC. Both Bernie and myself were adamantly opposed to acquiring this technology, which seemed noncompetitive with that of Cerus. John's rationale, however, was different than ours and focused on the apparent readiness of the Pentose process for clinical studies. In addition, there could have been some personal reasons, such as getting rid of Bernie, with whom he had a thorny relationship.

To hedge our bets I decided to embark on a parallel development path. Together with a chemist, Ionel Rosenthal, with whom I had a long-term collaboration experience and who was spending a sabbatical year at Vitex, we initiated studies of a very short-lived alkylating agent. The selectivity of this chemical derived from its rapid decomposition in water on one hand, and the ability of the chemical that reacted with nucleic acids, forming monoadducts to continue reacting to form nucleic acid crosslinks. The latter are very lethal to viruses. The approach resulted in promising early results but we did not have enough time to bring it to a stage that will impact Vitex's future.

Things came to a head during a Vitex board meeting in mid 1999, when the board decided to acquire Pentose in a stock swap deal. A few months later there was a reorganization of the company when Bernie was absent on a trip. Most of the RCC group, including myself, and some others in the R&D department were fired. Bernie has resigned as head of R&D a couple of months later and shortly thereafter the whole R&D operation was moved to Boston where Pentose was located. Almost all the remaining R&D personnel were let go on this occasion.

The reconfigured Vitex did enter clinical studies using the Pentose process for pathogen reduction in RCC. Those studies progressed into phase III despite the need for a few hours wash of the RCC following 24 hours of treatment. The studies were terminated when some of the treated patients developed antibodies against the treated red cells. Prior to that event Vitex sold its plasma operation to finance the clinical studies. When those failed it merged with another company, Panacos, that was developing a drug against HIV. Shortly thereafter Vitex ceased to exist even in name and John Barr was replaced as CEO. It is worthy of note that Cerus encountered the same problem as Vitex did during phase III. Cerus, however, was able to modify its process to prevent antibodies formation and had restarted a phase I clinical study.

The Vitex personnel fired, including myself, were in a state of shock even though we knew something was brewing. Fortunately, I was offered 4 months severance pay and access to the office of a placement company during this period. After some fruitless efforts at finding an appropriate position, in part because of my age at the time (59), I decided to be self-employed. I launched myself as a consultant to companies in the blood business. The results of this decision will be described in the coming chapters.

CHAPTER 14

POSTMORTEM

T HE MAJOR REASON for the failure of Vitex as a commercial enterprise lies in its inability to get a significant market share for its product, SD-plasma. Some of the reasons for this failure were alluded to before but a more in depth analysis will be useful.

One of the main reasons was the recalcitrance of blood banks to embrace virus inactivation in addition to testing. This reluctance was in spite of the obvious benefit of eliminating the risk of transmission of HIV, HBV and HCV. Even more important was the elimination of the risk of emerging viruses, and WNV is a case in point. The blood centers based their reluctance on the perceived risk of a pooled blood component and the added cost. More likely, conservatism and political reasons (such as the rivalry between the blood centers and ARC) played a major role. This experience was in stark contrast to the situation in Europe, where SD-plasma was universally adopted. Timing was a major factor too. SD-plasma became available in Europe around 1990, when the lessons of HIV emergence were still fresh and many governments mandated the use of virus-inactivated plasma.

The demand by FDA (which was supported by the blood banking community) that Vitex satisfy the entire market demand upon launch of SD-plasma put a considerable logistical and financial strains on the company. This stipulation was driven by fear of lawsuits by people infected after use of non-sterilized plasma. As a result, Vitex had to have the costly capacity to satisfy the demand of whole US market while using only about 10% of this capacity.

Another contributing factor was that none of the products in the pipeline became commercially available. This by itself would have been tolerable had SD-plasma been a commercial success.

Finally, the clash of personalities between John Barr, the CEO, and Bernie, did not help matters. John was abrasive, and while he had some prior experience in the blood industry he was no match to Bernie in terms of understanding all the scientific and political underpinnings of the blood business. Still, John tried to exert control and was instrumental in causing Bernie to leave at the end.

CHAPTER 15

A NEW ERA

THE FIRST STEP I took upon deciding on becoming a consultant was preparing a list of the companies, including a contact person within each company, that may be interested in my services. The list contained some 30 names with whom I was personally acquainted. I then sent a standard letter to each, letting them know my new circumstances and my availability as a consultant for blood safety in general and pathogen reduction in blood in particular. While the response was not overwhelming, over the next few months there were a few, two of them proving pivotal in keeping me in business.

The new period in my life coincided with a physical move of my lodgings. Since I was no longer an employee of the NYBC I had to vacate their apartment on the east side of Manhattan. The Vitex facility was located on the west side so we looked for an apartment on the upper west side to cut on commuting time. We found a reasonable apartment in the vicinity of Lincoln Center. The nearness to the Metropolitan Opera, the bustle of the area and proximity to great food resources made the change attractive. Luckily the housing market boom was just starting and the apartment was affordable. After the upheaval at Vitex we settled down to a less hectic pace and I began to enjoy more of the ample cultural offerings at the big apple.

In early 2000 I heard from a number of sources with regard to consulting on a number of projects. In addition to the main ones, to be discussed later, there were some projects of a limited nature. Because of non-disclosure agreements the companies cannot be identified. One company asked me to evaluate options to incorporate a pathogen reduction step for their plasma operations. This project took a few weeks and involved a visit to their facility to make a presentation and discuss recommendations. The company decided not to pursue this option so there was no follow-up. Another project was similar in nature, but more practical, involving the implementation of a pathogen reduction step in the manufacturing process of a biological product. Over time there were a number of additional minor projects, which took a small part of my time but supplied some income and kept me on my mental toes. One of them was of particular interest since it involved a novel process for long-term preservation of red cells. Unfortunately, this cannot be discussed at this time. And now, to the main attractions.

CHAPTER 16

PHOTOBIOCHEM

URING THE COURSE of my work at NYBC and Vitex I kept in contact with Dr Tom Dubbelman at Leiden University. After I left his lab when my sabbatical with him was over toward the end of 1991, he took on a doctoral student to continue my work on the mechanism of action of PDT. I served as an advisor for her thesis and visited the lab on a yearly basis. Later, another doctoral student was added, to work on the use of Pc for pathogen reduction in red cells. Naturally, as the world expert on the subject she was added to my advisory responsibilities. Meantime, Tom's lab in collaboration with the Netherlands Central Blood Bank, started looking at other potential photosensitizers for use in pathogen reduction in red cell concentrates.

About the time I left Vitex, the interest of Leiden University in supporting PDT research was waning and Tom decided to shift his efforts towards commercial applications. He accepted an offer from Boston Clinics, a private company involved with lasers in dermatology, to be the chief scientific officer of a spin-off—Boston Clinics PDT. The purpose of the spin-off was to develop PDT applications for dermatology. In 2000 Boston Clinics stopped its operation in Leiden as well as the financing of the spin-off. Tom and the CEO of Boston Clinics PDT, Dr Richard Stokvis, decided then to change direction. They renamed the company Photobiochem and focused on pathogen reduction in blood. By then Tom identified a positively charged porphyrin molecule that seemed to be able to efficiently kill viruses in RCC when exposed to red light, without undue damage to the red cells. He patented the molecule (termed Sylsens) and collaborated with the blood bank and University of Leiden to further develop the process. When he heard of my new situation he asked me to serve as a consultant to the new company—Photobiochem. I agreed enthusiastically and we settled on a compensation that would start as soon as funds were raised for the new company. Dr Stokvis (the CEO), a jovial and energetic fellow, addressed the funding effort head-on and in short order raised over $1M from Johnson and

Johnson Development arm and private investors to commence operations. These were actually done at Tom's lab at the university, which was now funded mostly by the company. The lab activities were focused on pathogen reduction on the one hand and collateral damage to red cells on the other. In addition, there were efforts to optimize the treatment conditions.

My role was on two fronts. First, I had to review their efforts and suggest modifications. Second, I had to come up with a prototype device for the scale-up from the lab scale treatment of a few ml of blood to a full red cell unit of 450 ml. For this purpose I contacted the engineering outfit in NJ that worked with me on scaling up the red cells process while in Vitex. We decided that the static mixing approach we came up with towards the end of my tenure at Vitex was the most appropriate. I then made the case to the company and after a lot of discussions and visits to the contractor Photobiochem agreed to pursue this approach.

Meanwhile, Richard decided to do a small-scale clinical study to demonstrate the feasibility of the process, the success of which would boost the funding efforts. The study was designed to show that the treated red cells circulated normally after infusion. The problem was that a prototype device was not yet ready and the treatment would be done in the lab under non-optimal conditions. I argued against such a shortcut as too risky, and so did Tom, but Richard went ahead anyway. The results of the study showed that the treated red cells' half-life in the circulation was reduced compared to untreated cells. While the reduction was not large it was enough to rule out the use of such treated cells for transfusion purposes and indicated that some improvement in the process was needed.

Because funding was inadequate and as a result additional studies to demonstrate that the process could be sufficiently improved were not done, this was a fatal blow for Photobiochem. Although the development of the prototype was accelerated and initial studies showed it to function as planned, money was in short supply to bring the necessary studies to conclusion before further funds could be raised. This was exacerbated by the decision of J&J to drop out of the picture. Some frantic efforts were made, the board of directors replaced the CEO with a more seasoned one, Dr Jaap Kampinga, but all was in vain. In 2004 the company was effectively closed, even though a salvage of the process was quite possible.

Tom returned to his university position but since funding was no longer available for PDT he took early retirement shortly thereafter. I was very sorry to see this wothwhile effort fizzle but by that time I was busy with another major effort.

DR. EHUD BEN-HUR

CHAPTER 17

ULTRAVIOLET BLOOD IRRADIATION

D URING THE 1930'S and 1940's a new treatment modality for infectious disease, both bacterial and viral, became popular. The process, ultraviolet blood irradiation (UBI), involved the drawing of a small volume of the patient's blood (about 250 ml) and passing it through the Knot's machine. The device was comprised of a broadband UV light source that was water-cooled and contained a flow cell through which the blood passed while being exposed to UV light. The treated blood was returned to the patient. The treatment was performed on an as needed basis, averaging 1-4 times over a period of a week to a few months. The rationale for the treatment was based on the germicidal property of UV light. The fact that only a small portion of the patient's blood was treated at any time ruled out inactivation of the pathogen as the sole underlying mechanism for the efficacy of the treatment. No controlled clinical studies were done at the time but the anecdotal reports of thousands of treated patients were generally positive. The treated patients recovered faster than could be expected.

The treatment never attained wider acceptance because of the cumbersome device and the lack of scientific understanding as to how it worked. When antibiotics became widely available UBI was abandoned. During the 1990's many pathogens became drug-resistant to commonly used antibiotics and some viral diseases, primarily those caused by HIV and HCV, became a serious health threat. This state of affairs raised the interest of some people in UBI. One of them was Thomas Petrie, an engineer with medical device experience.

I first met Tom in 1999, when he visited Vitex together with the VP of a small medical device company in which he worked at the time. The purpose of the meeting was to get Vitex interested in UBI and support the effort of bringing it to market again. Tom patented a new flow cell and a much more compact device to carry out UBI. Vitex did not express an interest in partnering to develop UBI and the matter rested there for a while.

In early 2000, when I became a consultant, I sent a letter to that effect to all my contacts in the industry, among them the above medical device company. They responded promptly and suggested we meet to discuss a consultancy agreement. The meeting was held with the VP and Tom, who were quite enthusiastic about me coming on board to help with their UBI project. To start the ball rolling they arranged a larger meeting, in which some physicians involved with UBI were also present. During that meeting the strategy to commercialize UBI was discussed, as well as the indication on which to focus initially. The easiest approach was to try to get a 510k approval for the device from the FDA. This kind of approval is based on the contention that the new device is basically the same as the Knott's machine.

Unfortunately, the FDA did not buy this argument. Their logic was that even assuming the two devices are basically the same, the Knot's machine never undergone double-blind clinical studies to demonstrate its efficacy and never received FDA approval at the time (it was commercialized before such approval was mandated by law). As a result, to get an approval UBI will have to go the hard way and demonstrate its efficacy and lack of side effects prior to commercialization. This route proved beyond the resources of the small device company and it dropped the project.

Tom, however, was adamant to continue to pursue UBI. He fervently believed this was a panacea and that the device he built has a place in the medical world.

CHAPTER 18

ENERGEX SYSTEMS

FORTUNATELY, SHORTLY AFTER he left the company to pursue UBI on his own, Tom met another Tom, Tom Fagan. The latter is an entrepreneur who had a prototype device to treat pain by short radiofrequency pulses. He asked Tom to join him and modify the device (later termed the Enrgex) in order to make it commercially acceptable. While discussing their arrangement Tom Petrie mentioned UBI and Fagan enthusiastically agreed that it would complement their new company pipeline of products. As a result, the new company, Energex Systems, Inc. was launched with Tom Fagan as the CEO and Tom Petrie as Director of Engineering. At this stage, and for some time to come, Energex was a virtual company with 3-4 employees. With the exception of the construction of the UBI device (christened the ImmunoModulator, or IM for short), all activities were outsourced. The company raised some money from private investors, did a clinical study with the Energex device that demonstrated its efficacy and got FDA approval to market it.

At this point, Tom Petrie asked me to renew our relationship and to help in guiding UBI through the studies needed to obtain FDA approval. I agreed and we soon met to discuss our strategy. My take was that prior to entering a clinical study Energex will have to demonstrate the safety of the device in preclinical studies using animals. I devised protocols appropriate for this purpose. The studies were then carried out by contract laboratories. In addition, Tom approached a scientist at Tulane University who did some viral studies with the device on a collaborative basis. Those studies showed that during the passage of the blood through the IM device about 30% of the virus added to the blood was inactivated. The results of these studies supported the safety of the device. We sent the FDA a package containing all the pertinent information and asked for a meeting, termed a pre-IDE (Investigative Device Exemption). The purpose of this meeting was to present our device and the studies done so far in order to get FDA feedback and perspective on the proposed clinical studies. At the meeting

Tom Fagan summarized the results to-date. The FDA was represented by some 10 scientists and administrators. The participants had quite a few questions about the process. They asked for additional studies to address more safety issues. We proposed a study in HCV-infected patients and the FDA was intent on ensuring the safety of the patients. The other point of discussion was how to define efficacy and what would constitute the primary endpoint for the study. We suggested a reduction of 2/3 of the viral load to begin with in a pilot study involving 10 patients.

After completing the requested additional preclinical studies we submitted all the information to the FDA who then approved the initiation of the clinical pilot study. It was done at Warren Hospital, Phillipsburg, NJ. The patients were followed up for 3 months after treatment. The results of the study were encouraging. There were no adverse effects as a result of the treatment. Viremia (the number of virus particles in the blood) decreased by 67% to 96% in 6 of the patients. The reduction in viremia, however, was not permanent. It returned to its initial value 10 weeks after cessation of the treatments.

Energex then convened a meeting with immunologists and virologists to discuss the results and decide on the course of action. The consensus was that UBI was definitely effective in a number of patients. For the second study we decided on an additional course of treatment 3 months after the first one, to obtain a more lasting effect, with a follow up period of 6 months. The FDA agreed to our new treatment protocol for another cohort of 10 patients. However, in addition to following the patients' viremia they asked for a liver biopsy to be taken prior to and at the end of the follow up period.

The second clinical study took about a year to complete. Again the results were encouraging. Viremia went down in most of the patients and the reduction extended for a longer period than in the first study. While none of the patients was virus-free at the end of the follow up period, their liver biopsies showed a reduction in inflammation. This finding was very important since liver inflammation leads eventually to cirrhosis and loss of liver function.

Energex is now contemplating a pivotal study in order to obtain FDA approval for using the IM as a treatment for HCV patients. At the same time the Indian Health Ministry reviewed the results of these studies and is now in the process of approving the IM for routine treatment of HCV patients. If enough patients are treated under controlled conditions the FDA could consider the results when deciding to approve the IM for use in the US even in the absence of a pivotal study. Libya is also considering the adoption of the IM for treating HCV-infected patients.

CHAPTER 19

ADDITIONAL INDICATIONS FOR UBI TREATMENT

DURING THE COURSE of the clinical studies with HCV patients, Energex launched collaborative studies to identify additional indications for UBI treatment. One of the most important contemplated was the treatment of AIDS patients. Current drug therapy of AIDS is rather effective but it is not curative, it is expensive and has side effects. In addition, the high mutability of the virus is leading to the emergence of drug-resistant HIV strains.

In order to demonstrate the potential benefit of UBI treatment for AIDS patients, a study with three monkeys infected with simian immunodeficiency virus (SIV) was done at the primate center of Tulane University (LA). The monkeys were infected with SIV and after the acute stage of infection were treated seven times with the IM over three weeks.

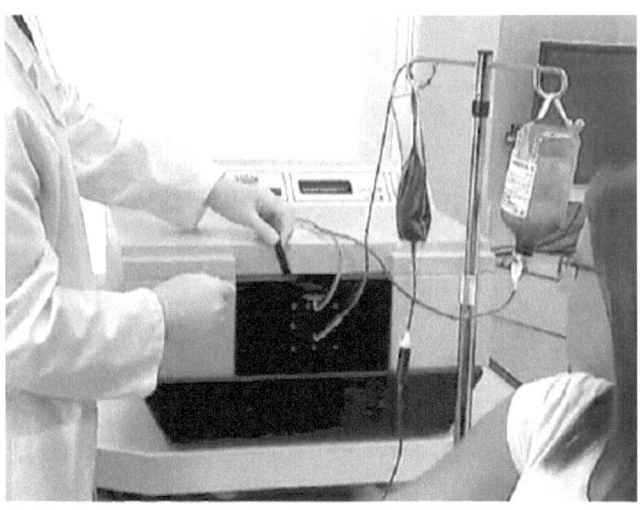

The ImmunoModulator in action,
courtesy of Energex Systems, Inc.

The results of this study were very encouraging. Two of the monkeys responded with a marked reduction of viremia. Parallel assays of immune parameters carried out on blood samples indicated a stimulation of the immune system in the two animals that responded to the treatment. In the animal that did not respond to the treatment stimulation of the immune system was not detected.

This study prompted the submission of an IDE request to the FDA to start a clinical study of AIDS patients. A meeting with the FDA was scheduled to discuss their concerns. I attended the meeting via the telephone. One of the main concerns raised by the FDA was related to cells that are latently infected with HIV. These cells serve as a pool of virus that is not affected by drug treatment and are the reason drug treatment against HIV infection is not curative. Exposure to UV light can activate HIV in latently infected cells. The activated virus then begins to proliferate in these cells. The FDA was concerned that the UBI treatment will activate the latent virus. I was asked to respond on behalf of Energex. My response was that such activation would benefit the patients. It would reduce the pool of hidden, untreatable virus. Moreover, the amount of new virus produced by the activation is only a small fraction of the total free HIV in the blood and would not materially affect viremia. It can be argued that depletion of the pool of latent virus by IM treatment, in conjunction with drug treatment, will allow a more effective therapy and even a potential cure if the pool of latent virus was sufficiently depleted.

The FDA granted approval to the proposed clinical study, in which reduced viremia and increase of CD4 cells are the primary endpoints. CD4 are the immune cells infected by HIV and their subsequent depletion results in the impairment of the immune system. Shortly thereafter a study of 10 AIDS patients was initiated and is ongoing. Preliminary results from the first two patients are encouraging. Following treatment, viremia was reduced and the number of CD4 cells in the blood increased significantly after treatment.

During the first clinical study of HCV patients one of the patients had a severe case of psoriasis. This is a skin disease that is thought to be autoimmune in origin. Following the treatment the psoriasis lesions have cleared. This raised the exciting possibility that UBI can ameliorate autoimmune diseases. A clinical study for treatment of psoriasis patients is currently being planned at the University of Alabama Medical Center in Birmingham.

DR. EHUD BEN-HUR

While Energex attention was focused on chronic viral infections such as HCV and HIV a new threat became apparent. This was bird flu that was threatening to become a flu pandemic, similar to the devastating one in 1918. While this threat has not materialized so far, Energex decided to do an animal study to test the potential of UBI to address it.

The animal model used for the study were mice infected with an influenza virus strain H1N1 (the 1918 flu pandemic strain and the more recent swine flu strain are of the same type). When infected with sufficient number of viruses the mice launched a very strong immune response that caused the animals to drown in their own fluids. The strong immune response is usually the cause of death in the case of bird flu and the 1918 flu pandemic. This was also the reason that the death rate among young people was higher than in older ones in 1918, the younger having a more robust immune response.

The results of the study were striking. Although viremia was not reduced in the treated animals, they looked much better and none of them died. The untreated infected mice looked worse and some of them died. Postmortem examination revealed that the latter displayed strong infiltration of the lungs by immune cells. This was not seen in the UBI-treated mice. Thus, the modulation of the immune response by UBI treatment can be beneficial in acute viral infections as well as chronic ones

While up to now studies of UBI were focused exclusively on treating infections and, more recently, autoimmune diseases, there is an untapped potential indication. The immune system is essential in controlling cancer, as evidenced from the high occurrence of the rare skin cancer, Kaposi's sarcoma, in AIDS patients. It is therefore conceivable that treatment with the IM will be beneficial for cancer patients. Indeed, when mice were implanted with breast cancer cells and then treated with IM the rate of tumor growth was significantly slowed. This opens a whole new field for using the IM, which Energex intends to pursue in the future.

EPILOGUE

WHILE ENERGEX IS still pursuing and exploring the potential of UBI and its mechanism of action it has also embarked on utilizing its expertise for pathogen reduction in blood for transfusion. Thus, Tom has developed a device that is able to irradiate a very thin film of red cell concentrate with UV light. The device has undergone a couple of modifications after field tests. The current version (see picture below) is about to be tested again. At NYBC I explored this possibility by UV-irradiating red cell concentrate that has been diluted 50-fold in a flow cell. The results indicated that pathogen reduction was feasible under these conditions. I did not pursue this further since it was not practical to concentrate the red cells back. The new approach obviates this problem and may offer a simple and effective way to finally obtain a safer red cells concentrate for transfusion.

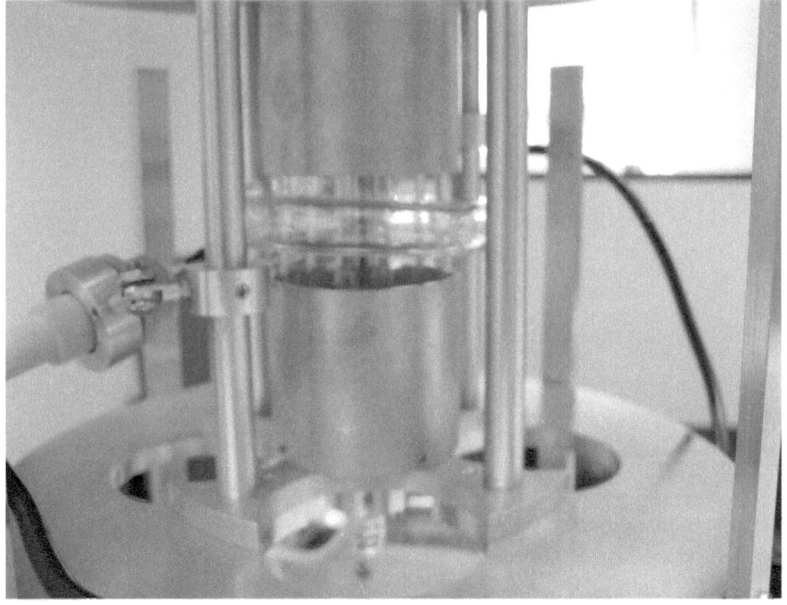

A prototype of a device for pathogen reduction
in RCC using UV light.
Courtesy of Energex Systems, Inc.

On a personal note, in 2005 my son Asa has accepted a position as an Assistant Professor at the Computer Science Department, Colorado State University (CSU) in Fort Collins. We spent a year there in 1983 on a sabbatical and loved the place. In 2007 I became semi-retired and we decided to move from NY to Fort Collins. We don't regret the move. We love that great little city, the laid back life style and recreational opportunities of the marvelous area. We visit NY frequently to recharge our cultural batteries and see our younger son, Adi. I usually meet with Tom Petrie on such occasions to discuss the latest scientific developments underlying the business of Energex.

GLOSSARY

AMT. A positively charged psoralen with a high affinity to nucleic acids. It is a very effective photosensitizer.

Amotosalen. A psoralen similar to AMT but even more effective and having less side effects, thus more suitable for pathogen reduction in blood.

Antibodies. Proteins produced by B lymphocytes against invading pathogens. They bind to the pathogens and help the immune system neutralize them.

Antioxidants. Chemicals that neutralize reactive oxygen species, thus preventing their deleterious effects.

ARC. American Red Cross, the emergency relief organization of the USA. Provides blood collection services and supplies about half the nation needs of blood for transfusion.

Blood groups. There are a number of specific sugars on the red cells that are immunogenic, resulting in production of antibodies when transfused into a recipient of a different group. The major ones are A and B. The AB group possess both and O lacks both. As a result, O is a universal donor.

Carnitine. A small molecule that is abundant in red cells and helps maintain the integrity of their membrane.

Cerus. The Cerus Corporation is the pioneer in developing processes for pathogen reduction in cellular components of blood. It currently provides a process for platelets concentrates and is conducting clinical studies for a process to treat red cells concentrates.

Chagas disease. The causative agent is a parasite, Trypanosoma cruzi, that is endemic in Latin America. Can be transmitted by blood transfusion because it is chronic and asymptomatic for many years.

Cryopharm. Cryopharm was launched in the early 1990's first to develop a process to store frozen platelets for transfusion and then to develop a process for pathogen reduction in platelets. None of these projects reached a fruition and the company declared bankruptcy in 1996.

Energex Systems, Inc. Energex was formed in 2000. Initially it developed and commercialized the Energex, a radiofrequency-emitting device for pain relief. It then started developing the ImmunoModulator, a device for UV blood-irradiation. The device is in clinical studies for the treatment of patients infected with HCV and HIV.

Erythrocytes. Red blood cells, lack a nucleus and possess a unique discoid shape. Their main function is to deliver oxygen from the lungs to body tissues.

Fibrin glue. When the blood protein fibrinogen is mixed with the clotting protein thrombin the latter splits the former into fibrin. Fibrin fibers are the main mass of a blood clot. When the two proteins are mixed over an open wound such as in surgery bleeding is stopped.

FFP. Fresh-frozen plasma, a blood component stored frozen. Used for transfusion in patients with clotting disorders.

Gambro. A Swedish company involved in the blood business. Its Navigent Biotechnology subsidiary in Denver, CO is developing a process for pathogen reduction in platelet concentrates based on riboflavin and termed Mirasol.

HAV. Hepatitis A virus, the causative agent of an acute liver disease. A small, non-lipid enveloped virus that is difficult to inactivate.

HBV. Hepatitis B virus, the causative agent of a chronic liver disease. Endemic in the Far East. Transmitted by blood transfusion. Lipid-enveloped. A vaccine is available.

HCV. Hepatitis C virus, the causative agent of a chronic liver disease. Transmitted by blood transfusion. Lipid-enveloped. No vaccine is available. About 4 million carriers in the USA. The disease can be cured by drugs in about 40-50% of patients. The treatment can take a year and involves side effects.

HIV. Human immunodeficiency virus, the causative agent of AIDS. A chronic disease that is incurable and there is no vaccine. Transmitted by blood transfusion, unprotected sex and reused needles for injection. Death is due to destroying of CD4 lymphocytes by the virus, a crucial element of the immune system. The patient subsequently succumbs to opportunistic microbes.

Hemoglobin. This is the oxygen carrier in red cells. Composed of globin (a protein made of 4 subunits) and heme. The latter is a porphyrin with an iron atom at its center to which the oxygen binds. Heme has a pronounced absorption of light in the blue, hence its intense red color.

HTLV. Human T lymphocytic virus, a retrovirus similar to HIV. Infects T lymphocytes chronically and can lead to leukemia. Transmitted by blood transfusion.

Inactines. Small, positively charged alkylating agents with affinity to nucleic acids. Upon binding they react covalently with the guanine base of nucleic acids and inactivates its function.

Leukoreduction. The process of filtering blood through filters that specifically retain the leukocytes. The most effective such filters can reduce the number of leukocytes in the blood by 6 logs.

Liposomes. Very small (50-500 nm) lipid vesicles that are used as special delivery vehicles for drugs.

Mad cow disease. A uniformly fatal disease of the brain. The causative agent is a protein called prion whose normal structure has been modified. The modified, abnormal prion molecules can induce normal prions to change their conformation. The abnormal prions are insoluble, accumulate in brain cells and destroy them.

Methylene blue. A phenothiazine dye with affinity to nucleic acids. Absorbs strongly red light hence its blue color. Serves as a photosensitizer by producing reactive oxygen species upon light exposure. These react with the guanine base of nucleic acids and inactivate their function.

NAT. Nucleic acid technology, a very sensitive technology used to detect nucleic acids by an amplification process. Can detect as low as 10 molecules in a sample.

Nanofiltration. The use of filters with pores small enough (20-60 nm) to exclude most viruses.

Parvovirus B 19. A small non-lipid enveloped virus that causes red cell hemolysis. Can be transmitted by blood transfusion. Poses a danger to pregnant women and patients with compromised immune system.

Pathogen reduction. A process designed to reduce the levels of pathogens in a biological sample by at least 7 logs. The purpose of the process is to increase the safety when transfusing or transplanting the sample to a patient with respect to transmission of infectious diseases.

Pc. Phthalocyanines are porphyrin-like molecules with intense absorption of red light and deep blue color. Used a lot in industry as pigments. Some of them are very effective photosensitizers that produce reactive oxygen species upon exposure to red light.

PDT. Photodynamic treatment is a procedure by which pathological lesions such as cancer are treated by a photosensitizer dye that localizes in the lesion, followed by light exposure that causes destruction of that lesion.

Pentose. A biotech company formed in the 1990's to develop the inactines as a process for pathogen reduction in RCC.

Photobiochem. A biotech company formed in 2002 by Richard Stokvis and Tom Dubbelman to develop a porphyrin as a photosensitizer for pathogen reduction in RCC.

Photosensitizer. A dye molecule that can transfer the light energy it absorbs to another molecule such as oxygen, resulting in chemical reactions.

Plasma. Plasma is the blood component left after the removal of red cells and platelets.

Porphyrin. A class of molecules composed of 4 pyrole molecules fused as a ring by carbon bridges. Serve many functions in biochemical processes. Absorb blue light strongly, hence their red color.

Psoralens. Chemicals found in some foodstuffs that bind in the dark to nucleic acids and form covalent bonds with the nucleic acid pyrimidines upon exposure to UVA light. As a result the nucleic acid is inactivated.

Psoriasis. Skin condition in which there is excess proliferation of the skin cells, resulting in red looking skin with scales. While the cause is not clear there is an involvement of the immune system and it appears to be an autoimmune disease.

RCC. Red cell concentrate, a blood component used for transfusion obtained by removing the plasma and platelets by centrifuging whole blood.

Riboflavin. A chemical that belongs to the B vitamin group. Has an affinity to nucleic acids and serves as a photosensitizer by producing reactive oxygen species when exposed to blue light.

SD-plasma. FFP that is pooled and treated with a solvent and detergent to inactivate lipid-enveloped viruses. The chemicals are then removed by affinity chromatography.

UBI. UV blood-irradiation, a process in which a portion of a patient's blood is exposed to UV light and is then returned to the patient. Used for the treatment of chronic viral infections. UBI appears to work by modulating the response of immune system.

UV light. Ultraviolet light is the portion of the electromagnetic spectrum beyond the violet of the visual portion (180-380 nm). Further divided into UVA (320-380 nm), UVB (290-320 nm) and UVC (180-290 nm). The UVC is absorbed by the ozone in earth atmosphere and does not reach the earth surface. This is the most deleterious of the UV light.

Viremia. The presence of virus particles in the blood.

Vitex. VI Technologies, Inc. was a biotech company spun-off by the New York Blood Center to commercialize some products developed at NYBC. In particular it focused on pathogen reduction in blood for transfusion.

Vitiligo. A skin disorder in which patches of skin lack pigmentation.

West Nile Virus. A lipid-enveloped virus that causes usually mild flu-like symptoms but can cause in some cases severe neurological complications and even death. The vector is a mosquito but the virus can also be transmitted by blood transfusion. Appeared in the USA in early 2000 in NY and spread to the whole country. Prevalence goes down as more of the population becomes immune due to infection.

White blood cells. This is the cellular part of the immune system (some immune cells are also present in the skin and gut). The most important are the T lymphocytes (produced in the thymus) and the B lymphocytes (produced in the bone marrow). The latter are responsible for production of antibodies.